FLEX AND THRIVE

A Step-by-Step Plan for Knee Joint Pain Recovery

DEVARAJAN PILLAI G

PREFACE

Welcome to "Flex and Thrive: A Step-by-Step Plan for Knee Joint Pain Recovery." If you've picked up this book, chances are you're no stranger to the discomfort and limitations that knee joint pain can bring to your life. Whether you're an athlete recovering from an injury, someone dealing with chronic pain, or simply seeking preventive measures, this book is crafted to be your guide on the journey to renewed knee health.

The human knee is an intricate joint, and when it's compromised, it can significantly impact your daily activities and overall well-being. As someone who has experienced the challenges of knee pain firsthand, I understand the frustration, the setbacks, and the desire for effective solutions.

"Flex and Thrive" is not just another self-help book; it's a comprehensive and practical resource designed to empower you with knowledge, strategies, and a step-by-step plan for reclaiming a pain-free and active lifestyle. Throughout these pages, you will find a blend of medical insights, holistic approaches, and actionable exercises aimed at addressing the root causes of knee joint pain.

This book is not a quick fix but a holistic journey towards recovery. It combines evidence-based information with real-life success stories, offering you a roadmap to navigate the complexities of knee health. From understanding the anatomy of the knee to implementing targeted exercises and lifestyle adjustments, each chapter is meticulously crafted to provide you with the tools you need to flex your way to thriving knees.

Remember, healing is a process, and this book is your companion on that journey. As you embark on this path to recovery, approach it with patience, commitment, and the belief that you have the capacity to regain control of your knee health.

May "Flex and Thrive" be a source of inspiration, knowledge, and empowerment on your quest for pain-free and flexible knees. Here's to a future where you not only manage knee joint pain but overcome it and emerge stronger than ever.

Wishing you a flexible and thriving journey ahead.

Warm regards,

DEVARAJAN PILLAI G

COPYRIGHT WARNING

DISCLAIMER

The information provided in this book, "Flex and Thrive: A Step-by-Step Plan for Knee Joint Pain Recovery," is intended for general informational purposes only. It is not a substitute for professional medical advice, diagnosis, or treatment. Always seek the advice of your physician or qualified healthcare provider with any questions you may have regarding a medical condition. The author and the publisher of this book are not medical professionals, and the content within these pages is based on research, personal experiences, and general knowledge up to the knowledge cutoff date of January 2022. While efforts have been made to ensure the accuracy and completeness of the information presented, medical knowledge is constantly evolving, and new developments may impact the recommendations provided.

Individual responses to the strategies, exercises, and recommendations outlined in this book may vary. It is crucial to consult with a healthcare professional before beginning any new exercise or treatment program, especially if you have pre-existing health conditions or concerns.

The author and the publisher disclaim any liability or responsibility for any loss, injury, or damage incurred as a direct or indirect consequence of the use or application of any information presented in this book. The reader assumes full responsibility for their actions and should use their discretion in applying the advice within this book to their specific circumstances.

Furthermore, any mention of specific products, treatments, or services in this book does not constitute an endorsement. Readers are encouraged to conduct their own research and consult with qualified healthcare professionals before making decisions about their health.

By reading this book, you acknowledge and agree to the terms of this disclaimer. If you do not agree with these terms, you should not use the information provided in this book or follow the suggested recommendations.

Thank you for your understanding.

DEVARAJAN PILLAI G

CONTENTS

1. UNDERSTANDING KNEE ANATOMY

The Foundation for Recovery

The human knee is a marvel of engineering, a complex joint that plays a crucial role in our daily movements. However, for many individuals, knee joint pain can disrupt the harmony of this intricate structure, leading to discomfort and limitations. In "Flex and Thrive: A Step-by-Step Plan for Knee Joint Pain Recovery," understanding the anatomy of the knee serves as the foundational key to unlocking the secrets of effective recovery. In this chapter, we delve into the intricacies of knee anatomy, exploring the components that contribute to its function and the common issues that can lead to pain.

The Anatomy of the Knee

The knee joint is a hinge joint connecting the thigh bone (femur) to the shinbone (tibia). The kneecap (patella) glides along the front of the femur in a groove, adding stability to the joint. Ligaments, which are tough bands of connective tissue, hold the bones together, providing stability and preventing excessive movement. Meanwhile, the muscles surrounding the knee contribute to its movement and support.

Key Components of Knee Anatomy:

1. **Bones:**
   - Femur (Thigh Bone)
   - Tibia (Shinbone)

- Patella (Kneecap)
- Fibula (Smaller Bone beside Tibia)

2. **Ligaments:**
   - Anterior Cruciate Ligament (ACL)
   - Posterior Cruciate Ligament (PCL)
   - Medial Collateral Ligament (MCL)
   - Lateral Collateral Ligament (LCL)

3. **Cartilage:**
   - Meniscus (Medial and Lateral)

4. **Muscles:**
   - Quadriceps
   - Hamstrings
   - Calf Muscles

Understanding the Function

The knee is a weight-bearing joint responsible for a range of movements, including flexion (bending), extension (straightening), and limited rotation. These movements are facilitated by the coordinated action of muscles, ligaments, and tendons.

1. **Ligaments and Stability:**
   - ACL and PCL prevent excessive forward and backward movement.
   - MCL and LCL provide stability on the inner and outer sides of the knee.

2. **Meniscus and Cushioning:**
   - The meniscus acts as a shock absorber, providing cushioning between the femur and tibia.

3. **Muscles and Movement:**
   - Quadriceps muscles straighten the knee.
   - Hamstrings muscles bend the knee.

Common Issues Affecting Knee Anatomy

Understanding the knee's anatomy is crucial in identifying the root causes of pain and dysfunction. Several common issues can impact the knee joint:

1. **Osteoarthritis:**

- Gradual wear and tear of cartilage.
2. **Tendonitis:**
   - Inflammation of tendons, often due to overuse.
3. **Ligament Tears:**
   - ACL, PCL, MCL, or LCL injuries can result from sudden twists or impacts.
4. **Meniscus Tears:**
   - Tears in the meniscus can occur due to sudden movements or degeneration.
5. **Bursitis:**
   - Inflammation of fluid-filled sacs (bursae) around the knee.
6. **Patellar Tracking Issues:**
   - Misalignment of the kneecap.

Understanding these issues sets the stage for developing a targeted recovery plan, tailored to address specific challenges and promote overall knee health.

Recovery Strategies Based on Anatomy

Recovering from knee joint pain involves addressing the underlying causes and promoting the health of each component. Here's a breakdown of strategies based on knee anatomy:

1. **Strengthening Muscles:**
   - Targeting quadriceps, hamstrings, and calf muscles to provide better support to the knee joint.
2. **Balancing Flexibility and Stability:**
   - Incorporating exercises that enhance flexibility without compromising joint stability.
3. **Low-Impact Cardiovascular Exercise:**
   - Engaging in activities like swimming or cycling to promote cardiovascular health without excessive impact on the knee joint.
4. **Nutrition for Joint Health:**
   - Adopting a diet rich in nutrients that support joint health, including omega-3 fatty acids and antioxidants.

5. **Mind-Body Connection:**
    - Recognizing the influence of mental well-being on physical recovery and incorporating mindfulness practices.

2.DEMYSTIFYING JOINT PAIN

Common Causes and Triggers

Joint pain can be an unwelcome companion, disrupting our daily lives and hindering our ability to move freely. In the quest for knee joint pain recovery outlined in "Flex and Thrive: A Step-by-Step Plan for Knee Joint Pain Recovery," it is crucial to demystify the origins of joint pain. Understanding the common causes and triggers is the first step toward creating an effective and personalized recovery plan. In this chapter, we unravel the mysteries surrounding joint pain, exploring the factors that contribute to discomfort and limitations.

The Complexity of Joint Pain

Joint pain is a complex phenomenon influenced by various factors, including genetics, lifestyle, and overall health. While the focus here is on knee joint pain, it's essential to recognize that joint pain can manifest in different areas of the body, and the principles discussed can be applied broadly.

1. **Inflammatory Conditions:**
   - Rheumatoid arthritis, osteoarthritis, and gout are examples of inflammatory joint conditions. In these cases, the immune system may mistakenly attack the joints, leading to pain, swelling, and stiffness.
2. **Overuse and Wear-and-Tear:**

- Repetitive stress on a joint, often due to activities like running or high-impact sports, can lead to overuse injuries. Over time, wear-and-tear on the joints can contribute to pain and inflammation.

3. **Trauma and Injuries:**
   - Accidents, falls, or sports injuries can result in trauma to the joints, causing immediate pain or contributing to chronic issues over time.

4. **Age-Related Changes:**
   - As we age, the cartilage that cushions our joints may wear down, leading to conditions like osteoarthritis. Changes in bone density and muscle mass can also impact joint health.

5. **Genetic Factors:**
   - Some individuals may be predisposed to joint issues due to genetic factors. Understanding family history can provide insights into potential risks.

6. **Obesity:**
   - Excess weight puts additional stress on weight-bearing joints, such as the knees. This can contribute to the development or exacerbation of joint pain.

Common Causes of Knee Joint Pain

Now, let's delve into the specific causes of knee joint pain, shedding light on the common culprits that may be behind your discomfort:

1. **Osteoarthritis:**
   - The most prevalent form of arthritis, osteoarthritis occurs when the protective cartilage that cushions the ends of bones wears down over time. This can lead to pain, swelling, and reduced joint mobility.

2. **Rheumatoid Arthritis:**
   - An autoimmune disorder where the immune system mistakenly attacks the synovium, the lining of the membranes that surround the joints. This can result in inflammation, pain, and joint deformities.

3. **Meniscus Tears:**

- The meniscus is a wedge-shaped cartilage in the knee that acts as a cushion between the femur and tibia. Tears in the meniscus can occur due to sudden twists, impacting the knee's ability to absorb shock.

4. **Ligament Injuries:**
   - Injuries to the ACL (anterior cruciate ligament) or other ligaments can cause instability and pain in the knee.

5. **Bursitis:**
   - Inflammation of the bursae, small fluid-filled sacs that cushion the outside of the knee joint. Bursitis can result from overuse or repeated pressure on the knee.

6. **Patellofemoral Pain Syndrome:**
   - Also known as runner's knee, this condition involves pain around the kneecap and is often associated with overuse or misalignment of the patella.

7. **Gout:**
   - A form of arthritis caused by the accumulation of uric acid crystals in the joints, leading to sudden and severe pain.

Identifying Triggers for Joint Pain

Understanding the causes of knee joint pain is just the beginning. Identifying triggers that exacerbate pain or contribute to flare-ups is equally important in developing an effective recovery plan:

1. **Poor Posture and Body Mechanics:**
   - Incorrect body mechanics during activities can put unnecessary stress on the knee joint. Addressing posture and movement patterns is essential for joint health.

2. **Inactivity and Sedentary Lifestyle:**
   - Lack of physical activity can contribute to muscle weakness and joint stiffness. Conversely, excessive sedentary behavior can also be detrimental to joint health.

3. **Improper Footwear:**
   - Wearing shoes with inadequate support or an improper fit can impact the alignment of the lower body, leading to knee pain.
4. **Unmanaged Stress:**
   - Chronic stress can contribute to inflammation and exacerbate symptoms of inflammatory joint conditions.
5. **Weather Changes:**
   - Some individuals report increased joint pain during changes in weather, although the scientific evidence on this connection is inconclusive.
6. **Dietary Choices:**
   - Certain foods, especially those high in purines, can trigger gout attacks. Maintaining a balanced and anti-inflammatory diet is crucial.
7. **Excessive Weight:**
   - Carrying excess weight places additional stress on weight-bearing joints. Achieving and maintaining a healthy weight is beneficial for joint health.

Developing a Personalized Recovery Plan

As we demystify joint pain and uncover its causes and triggers, the path to recovery becomes clearer. "Flex and Thrive" provides a step-by-step plan that considers the unique factors contributing to your knee joint pain. Here are key strategies to include in your personalized recovery plan:

1. **Medical Evaluation:**
   - Consult with a healthcare professional to accurately diagnose the underlying cause of your knee joint pain.
2. **Targeted Exercises:**
   - Engage in exercises that strengthen the muscles supporting the knee and improve flexibility. A physical therapist can provide a customized exercise plan.
3. **Weight Management:**

- If applicable, work towards achieving and maintaining a healthy weight to reduce stress on the knee joint.

4. **Joint-Friendly Nutrition:**
   - Adopt an anti-inflammatory diet rich in fruits, vegetables, whole grains, and omega-3 fatty acids.

5. **Proper Footwear:**
   - Invest in supportive footwear that promotes proper alignment and reduces strain on the knees.

6. **Posture and Body Mechanics:**
   - Address poor posture and incorrect body mechanics through awareness and corrective exercises.

7. **Stress Management:**
   - Incorporate stress-reducing practices such as mindfulness, meditation, or yoga to promote overall well-being.

3.ROAD TO RECOVERY

Setting Realistic Goals for Knee Health

Embarking on the road to recovery from knee joint pain is a transformative journey that requires not only dedication but a strategic plan that sets the stage for success. In "Flex and Thrive: A Step-by-Step Plan for Knee Joint Pain Recovery," understanding the importance of setting realistic goals becomes paramount. This chapter serves as your guide to navigating the road to recovery, outlining the significance of establishing achievable milestones for optimal knee health. The Power of Setting Goals

Setting goals is a powerful tool that can propel us toward positive change, especially when it comes to recovering from knee joint pain. Goals provide direction, motivation, and a framework for measuring progress. In the context of knee health, setting realistic and attainable goals is crucial for creating a sustainable plan that aligns with your unique needs and abilities.

1. **Clarity of Purpose:**
   - Goals provide clarity regarding what you aim to achieve. Whether it's reducing pain, improving mobility, or building strength, clearly defined goals serve as a roadmap for your recovery journey.
2. **Motivation and Focus:**
   - Knowing that you have specific objectives to reach can be a powerful motivator. Goals keep you focused

on the steps you need to take, even on challenging days.

3. **Progress Tracking:**
   - Goals act as benchmarks for progress. Regularly assessing how far you've come allows you to celebrate achievements and make informed adjustments to your plan.

4. **Empowerment and Control:**
   - Setting goals empowers you to take an active role in your recovery. It gives you a sense of control over your journey, fostering a positive mindset that is integral to healing.

Understanding Realistic Goals for Knee Health

The key to successful goal-setting lies in establishing realistic and achievable targets. Unrealistic goals can lead to frustration and setbacks, while attainable goals create a positive cycle of accomplishment and motivation. Let's explore the components of setting realistic goals for knee health:

1. **Specificity:**
   - Clearly define your goals with specific details. Instead of a vague aim like "reduce pain," specify the target, such as "reduce knee pain during daily activities by 30% in the next six weeks."

2. **Measurability:**
   - Make your goals measurable to track progress objectively. Quantifiable metrics, such as the number of pain-free steps taken or increased range of motion, provide tangible evidence of improvement.

3. **Achievability:**
   - Ensure your goals are realistic and attainable within a given timeframe. Assess your current abilities, taking into account any physical limitations, and set goals that push you without overwhelming you.

4. **Relevance:**

- Align your goals with your overall recovery objectives. Consider how each goal contributes to your broader plan for knee health and addresses specific challenges you may be facing.

5. **Time-Bound:**
   - Establish a timeframe for achieving your goals. This adds a sense of urgency and prevents procrastination. However, be mindful of setting realistic timelines that allow for gradual progress.

6. **Adaptability:**
   - Recognize that your needs and capabilities may evolve throughout your recovery journey. Be willing to adapt your goals as necessary, ensuring they remain relevant to your current circumstances.

Roadmap to Recovery: A Step-by-Step Approach

Now that we understand the principles of realistic goal-setting for knee health, let's outline a step-by-step approach to crafting your roadmap to recovery:

Step 1: Self-Assessment and Reflection

Begin by assessing your current state of knee health. Reflect on your pain levels, mobility, and any specific challenges you're experiencing. This self-awareness forms the foundation for setting targeted and meaningful goals.

Step 2: Define Your Objectives

Identify the specific aspects of knee health you want to improve. Whether it's reducing pain, increasing flexibility, or enhancing overall strength, articulate your objectives with clarity.

Step 3: Break Down Goals into Milestones

Divide your overarching goals into smaller, manageable milestones. This approach not only makes the journey more achievable but also allows for a steady progression of success.

Step 4: Prioritize and Sequencing

Prioritize your goals based on their significance to your overall knee health. Consider sequencing them in a way that builds upon each achievement, creating a logical and progressive path to recovery.

Step 5: Consult with Healthcare Professionals

Seek guidance from healthcare professionals, such as physical therapists or orthopedic specialists, to ensure your goals align with your physical condition. Their expertise can provide valuable insights and help tailor your plan to your unique needs.

Step 6: Set Baseline Metrics

Establish baseline metrics for each goal, providing a starting point for measurement. This could include recording pain levels, tracking steps taken without discomfort, or noting the range of motion in your knee.

Step 7: Establish Timeframes

Assign realistic timeframes to each goal and milestone. Be mindful of your daily schedule, commitments, and the gradual nature of recovery. Setting achievable deadlines encourages consistent effort.

Step 8: Build in Flexibility

Recognize that setbacks or unexpected challenges may arise. Building flexibility into your plan allows for adjustments without compromising your overall trajectory. Adaptability is a key component of successful recovery.

Step 9: Monitor and Celebrate Progress

Regularly monitor your progress against established metrics. Celebrate even the smallest victories, as they contribute to the positive momentum of your journey. Acknowledge your efforts and perseverance.

Step 10: Evaluate and Adjust

Periodically evaluate your goals and their alignment with your evolving needs. If certain goals become less relevant or new challenges emerge, be open to adjusting your plan accordingly. The ability to adapt is a strength.

Case Studies: Realistic Goals in Action

To illustrate the impact of realistic goal-setting, let's explore two hypothetical case studies:

Case Study 1: John's Journey to Reduced Pain

Objective: To reduce knee pain during daily activities.

Milestones:

1. **Week 1-2:** Implement a daily stretching routine for 10 minutes.
2. **Week 3-4:** Increase water intake to improve joint lubrication.
3. **Week 5-6:** Introduce low-impact exercises, such as swimming or cycling, for 20 minutes, three times a week.
4. **Week 7-8:** Consult with a physical therapist to refine the exercise routine for optimal pain management.
5. **Week 9-12:** Gradually increase exercise intensity and duration based on professional guidance.

Case Study 2: Sarah's Flexibility and Strength Improvement

Objective: To enhance flexibility and strength for better knee support.

Milestones:

1. **Week 1-2:** Begin a daily routine of gentle yoga for 15 minutes.
2. **Week 3-4:** Incorporate bodyweight exercises, such as squats and lunges, to improve muscle strength.
3. **Week 5-6:** Attend a structured flexibility and strength training class twice a week.
4. **Week 7-8:** Assess progress and modify the routine based on individual comfort and feedback.
5. **Week 9-12:** Gradually increase the intensity and complexity of exercises, integrating resistance training for added strength.

4.HOLISTIC HEALING

Integrating Mind, Body, and Spirit in Recovery

In the pursuit of knee joint pain recovery, the concept of holistic healing emerges as a powerful approach that transcends traditional medical boundaries. "Flex and Thrive: A Step-by-Step Plan for Knee Joint Pain Recovery" recognizes the interconnectedness of mind, body, and spirit, highlighting the significance of embracing a holistic perspective in the recovery process. This chapter explores the integration of holistic healing principles, providing a comprehensive guide to nurturing overall well-being and achieving lasting knee health.

Understanding Holistic Healing

Holistic healing is rooted in the belief that optimal health is not solely the absence of illness but a dynamic state that encompasses physical, mental, emotional, and spiritual well-being. Rather than treating symptoms in isolation, holistic healing addresses the underlying imbalances that contribute to health challenges. In the context of knee joint pain recovery, embracing a holistic approach involves recognizing the intricate interplay between the mind, body, and spirit.

1. **Mind:**
   - The mental aspect of holistic healing involves cultivating a positive mindset, managing stress, and addressing any psychological factors that may impact physical well-being.

2. **Body:**
   - The physical component focuses on the health of the body, including nutrition, exercise, and targeted therapies that support the recovery of the knee joint and overall musculoskeletal system.

3. **Spirit:**
   - The spiritual dimension encompasses a sense of purpose, connection, and inner peace. It involves nurturing the spirit through practices that promote self-awareness, mindfulness, and alignment with one's values.

Integrating Mind, Body, and Spirit in Knee Joint Pain Recovery

Mind: The Power of Positive Thinking

1. **Mind-Body Connection:**
   - Research has demonstrated the powerful link between the mind and the body. Positive thinking can influence the release of neurotransmitters and hormones that contribute to overall well-being.

2. **Stress Management:**
   - Chronic stress can exacerbate knee joint pain. Mindfulness meditation, deep breathing exercises, and other stress-reducing techniques can be valuable tools in managing both stress and pain.

3. **Cognitive Behavioral Therapy (CBT):**
   - CBT is a therapeutic approach that addresses negative thought patterns and behaviors. It can be beneficial in managing the emotional impact of chronic pain.

4. **Visualization and Guided Imagery:**
   - Envisioning the healing process and positive outcomes through visualization can contribute to a more optimistic outlook and enhance the body's natural healing mechanisms.

Body: Nutritional Support and Physical Well-being

1. **Anti-Inflammatory Diet:**
   - Inflammation is a common factor in joint pain. Adopting an anti-inflammatory diet rich in fruits, vegetables, whole grains, and omega-3 fatty acids can support the reduction of inflammation.
2. **Hydration:**
   - Proper hydration is essential for joint health. Water helps lubricate the joints and supports the overall function of the musculoskeletal system.
3. **Exercise and Physical Therapy:**
   - Tailored exercises and physical therapy play a crucial role in knee joint pain recovery. Strengthening the muscles around the knee, improving flexibility, and enhancing overall fitness contribute to a holistic approach.
4. **Alternative Therapies:**
   - Modalities such as acupuncture, chiropractic care, and massage therapy can complement traditional approaches, providing additional avenues for pain relief and overall well-being.

Spirit: Cultivating Inner Harmony

1. **Mindfulness Practices:**
   - Engaging in mindfulness practices, such as meditation and yoga, fosters a deeper connection with the present moment, promoting inner peace and reducing stress.
2. **Purpose and Meaning:**
   - Finding purpose and meaning in one's life can contribute to a sense of fulfillment and overall well-being. This can be achieved through personal pursuits, hobbies, or contributing to the well-being of others.
3. **Connection with Nature:**
   - Spending time in nature has been linked to various health benefits, including reduced stress and

improved mood. Connecting with the natural world can nourish the spirit.

4. **Holistic Therapies:**
   - Some individuals find solace in holistic therapies such as energy healing, Reiki, or aromatherapy. These practices aim to balance the body's energy and promote a sense of harmony.

Case Study: Holistic Healing in Action

Let's explore a hypothetical case study to illustrate the integration of mind, body, and spirit in knee joint pain recovery:

Case Study: Emily's Journey to Holistic Healing

Emily, a 45-year-old professional, has been experiencing chronic knee joint pain due to a combination of osteoarthritis and overuse. Frustrated with conventional treatments that provided temporary relief, Emily decides to embrace a holistic approach to recovery.

Mind:

- *Emily practices daily mindfulness meditation to manage stress and cultivate a positive mindset.*
- *She incorporates cognitive behavioral therapy techniques to address negative thought patterns related to her pain.*
- *Visualization exercises help Emily envision a future of pain-free movement and flexibility.*

Body:

- *Emily adopts an anti-inflammatory diet, focusing on whole foods, and includes omega-3 supplements to support joint health.*
- *She engages in a tailored exercise routine that combines strengthening exercises for the muscles around the knee and low-impact cardiovascular activities.*
- *Emily explores acupuncture sessions to complement her physical therapy and promote overall well-being.*

Spirit:

- *Mindful walking in nature becomes a daily practice for Emily, providing a sense of peace and connection with the environment.*
- *She explores holistic therapies such as aromatherapy and Reiki to enhance her spiritual well-being.*
- *Contributing to a local community project gives Emily a sense of purpose and fulfillment.*

Over the course of several months, Emily experiences a transformative shift. Her pain levels decrease, and she discovers a newfound resilience and connection with her body. By embracing holistic healing, Emily not only addresses the physical aspects of knee joint pain but nurtures her overall well-being.

5. FUELLING YOUR FLEXIBILITY

Nutrition's Role in Joint Health

Flexibility is a crucial aspect of overall health and well-being, and joint health plays a pivotal role in achieving and maintaining flexibility. One of the key factors influencing joint health is nutrition. In this comprehensive guide, we will explore the intricate connection between nutrition and joint health, focusing on how a well-balanced diet can contribute to the prevention and recovery from knee joint pain. This information is part of a larger book titled "Flex and Thrive: A Step-by-Step Plan for Knee Joint Pain Recovery."

Understanding Joint Health:

Before delving into the relationship between nutrition and joint health, it is essential to understand the structure and function of joints. Joints are the points where two or more bones meet, allowing for movement and flexibility. In the case of the knee joint, it is a complex structure involving bones, cartilage, ligaments, and synovial fluid. The health of these components collectively determines the overall well-being of the joint.

Common Factors Contributing to Knee Joint Pain:

Several factors can contribute to knee joint pain, ranging from injuries and overuse to degenerative conditions like osteoarthritis. However, nutrition can play a significant role in either preventing or exacerbating these issues.

1. **Maintaining a Healthy Weight:** Excess body weight places additional stress on the knee joints, particularly the weight-bearing joints like the knees. A well-balanced diet that helps in weight management is crucial in preventing and alleviating knee joint pain.
2. **Anti-Inflammatory Diet:** Inflammation is a common factor in joint pain, and certain foods can either contribute to or mitigate inflammation. An anti-inflammatory diet rich in fruits, vegetables, whole grains, and omega-3 fatty acids can help reduce inflammation and promote joint health.
3. **Vitamins and Minerals:** Adequate intake of vitamins and minerals is essential for maintaining the health of bones and cartilage. Vitamin D, calcium, and magnesium are particularly important for bone health, while vitamin C plays a crucial role in collagen synthesis, important for joint structure.

Nutrition for Joint Health:

1. **Omega-3 Fatty Acids:** Omega-3 fatty acids, found in fatty fish like salmon, flaxseeds, and walnuts, have anti-inflammatory properties. Incorporating these into your diet can help reduce inflammation in the joints and promote overall joint health.
2. **Antioxidant-Rich Foods:** Antioxidants help combat oxidative stress, which can contribute to joint damage. Berries, leafy greens, and colorful vegetables are rich sources of antioxidants that can support joint health.
3. **Collagen-Rich Foods:** Collagen is a vital protein for the health of connective tissues, including joints. Bone broth, chicken, fish, and collagen supplements can contribute to maintaining the integrity of the joints.
4. **Calcium and Vitamin D:** Calcium is crucial for bone health, and vitamin D facilitates its absorption. Dairy products, leafy greens, and exposure to sunlight are essential for maintaining adequate levels of these nutrients.
5. **Turmeric and Ginger:** Both turmeric and ginger possess anti-inflammatory properties. Including them in your diet, either

through spices or teas, can help reduce inflammation and alleviate joint pain.

Lifestyle Factors:

While nutrition is a cornerstone of joint health, it is essential to consider other lifestyle factors that can complement a healthy diet:

1. **Regular Exercise:** Engaging in appropriate exercises, such as low-impact activities like swimming or cycling, can strengthen the muscles around the knee joint and improve overall joint stability.
2. **Hydration:** Staying adequately hydrated is crucial for maintaining the synovial fluid that lubricates the joints. Water is essential for overall joint function and can contribute to reducing stiffness.
3. **Moderation in Alcohol and Caffeine Consumption:** Excessive alcohol and caffeine intake can contribute to inflammation. Moderation in consumption is advisable for individuals seeking to improve joint health.

6.STEP-BY-STEP WARM-UP

and

Cool-down Routines for Resilient Knees

T he road to resilient and pain-free knees involves more than just targeted exercises and a balanced diet. An often underestimated but crucial aspect of knee joint health is the warm-up and cool-down routine. In this article, we will delve into the importance of warming up and cooling down for resilient knees and provide a step-by-step guide as part of the book titled "Flex and Thrive: A Step-by-Step Plan for Knee Joint Pain Recovery."

Understanding the Importance of Warm-up and Cool-down:

The knee joint is a complex structure that bears the brunt of our daily activities, whether it's walking, running, or climbing stairs. Warming up before engaging in physical activity and cooling down afterward are essential components of a comprehensive knee care routine. These routines not only prepare the body for the demands of exercise but also aid in recovery, reducing the risk of injuries and promoting overall joint resilience.

Warm-up Benefits:

1. **Increased Blood Flow:** Warming up gradually increases blood flow to the muscles and joints, delivering oxygen and nutrients. This prepares the muscles for the upcoming activity, reducing the risk of strains and injuries.
2. **Enhanced Joint Lubrication:** As the body warms up, synovial fluid production increases, lubricating the joints and reducing friction. This is especially crucial for the knee joint, which relies on smooth movements.
3. **Improved Flexibility and Range of Motion:** Warm-up exercises gently stretch the muscles and ligaments, enhancing flexibility and range of motion. This is vital for preventing undue stress on the knee joint during physical activity.

Cool-down Benefits:

1. **Facilitates Muscle Recovery:** Cooling down helps to gradually bring the heart rate and breathing back to normal, preventing sudden stops that can lead to dizziness. This gradual reduction in intensity supports muscle recovery.
2. **Prevents Blood Pooling:** After intense physical activity, blood can pool in the extremities. A proper cool-down routine helps prevent this by promoting gradual redistribution of blood throughout the body.
3. **Reduces Muscle Stiffness and Soreness:** Stretching during the cool-down phase helps prevent muscle stiffness and soreness by promoting flexibility and realigning muscle fibers.

Step-by-Step Warm-up Routine:

1. **Cardiovascular Exercise (5-10 minutes):** Start with light cardiovascular exercises such as brisk walking, cycling, or jumping jacks. This increases heart rate, promotes blood flow, and prepares the entire body for more intense activity.
2. **Dynamic Stretching (5 minutes):** Engage in dynamic stretches that target the major muscle groups involved in the activity. For knees, focus on leg swings, knee circles, and lunges. Dynamic stretching gradually increases flexibility and range of motion.

3. **Joint Mobilization (2-3 minutes):** Perform gentle joint mobilization exercises, including ankle circles and knee rotations. This helps improve joint mobility and lubrication, reducing the risk of stiffness.
4. **Specific Knee Warm-up (5 minutes):** Before engaging in activities that put additional stress on the knees, perform specific knee warm-up exercises. These may include leg extensions, leg curls, and mini squats. Focus on controlled movements to activate the muscles around the knee joint.

Step-by-Step Cool-down Routine:

1. **Low-Intensity Cardio (5-10 minutes):** Gradually reduce the intensity of your workout with low-impact cardiovascular exercises. This can include walking or slow cycling. This helps to bring the heart rate down gradually.
2. **Static Stretching (8-10 minutes):** Focus on static stretches that target the major muscle groups used during the workout. For knees, include stretches like quadriceps stretches, hamstring stretches, and calf stretches. Hold each stretch for 15-30 seconds, breathing deeply to promote relaxation.
3. **Foam Rolling (5 minutes):** Incorporate foam rolling to release any tension in the muscles and fascia. Concentrate on the thighs, calves, and IT band to alleviate muscle tightness around the knee joint.
4. **Hydration and Nutrition (Post-Workout):** Rehydrate with water and replenish your body with a balanced post-workout snack or meal. Proper nutrition supports muscle recovery and overall joint health.

Incorporating these Warm-up and Cool-down Routines into Your Routine:

1. **Consistency is Key:** Make warming up and cooling down a non-negotiable part of your exercise routine. Consistency is crucial for reaping the full benefits and preventing injuries.
2. **Adapt to Your Activity:** Tailor your warm-up and cool-down routines based on the specific activities you engage in. Whether

it's running, weightlifting, or yoga, ensure your warm-up and cool-down address the unique demands of the activity.

3. **Listen to Your Body:** Pay attention to how your body responds to different warm-up and cool-down exercises. If certain movements cause discomfort, consider modifying or seeking guidance from a healthcare professional.

4. **Progress Gradually:** As your fitness level improves, you can gradually increase the intensity and duration of your warm-up and cool-down routines. This progression supports the ongoing resilience of your knees.

7.STRENGTH WITHIN

Building Muscular Support for Joint Stability

The journey towards resilient and pain-free knees involves more than just addressing the symptoms; it requires a holistic approach that encompasses various aspects of joint health. One critical element often overlooked is the role of muscular support in providing stability to the knee joints. In this article, we will explore the significance of building muscular strength for joint stability, providing a step-by-step guide as part of the book "Flex and Thrive: A Step-by-Step Plan for Knee Joint Pain Recovery."

Understanding the Importance of Muscular Support:

The knee joint, being a hinge joint, is particularly vulnerable to stress and strain, especially during weight-bearing activities. The surrounding muscles play a pivotal role in providing support and stability to the knee. Weakness or imbalances in these muscles can contribute to joint instability, leading to pain and increased susceptibility to injuries. Building muscular strength not only aids in preventing knee issues but also supports recovery for those experiencing joint pain.

Key Muscles Involved in Knee Stability:

1. **Quadriceps:** The quadriceps, a group of four muscles at the front of the thigh, play a crucial role in extending the knee. Strengthening the quadriceps provides stability during activities like walking, running, and climbing stairs.

2. **Hamstrings:** The hamstrings, located at the back of the thigh, help in bending the knee. Balanced strength between the quadriceps and hamstrings is essential for overall knee joint stability.
3. **Gluteal Muscles:** The gluteal muscles, including the gluteus maximus, medius, and minimus, contribute to hip stability. Strong glutes help maintain proper alignment and reduce stress on the knees.
4. **Calf Muscles:** The calf muscles, comprising the gastrocnemius and soleus, provide support during activities like walking and running. They play a role in controlling movement and absorbing shock.

Step-by-Step Guide to Building Muscular Support for Knee Stability:

1. **Assessment of Current Strength and Flexibility:** Before embarking on a strength-building program, assess your current strength and flexibility levels. Identify any muscle imbalances or areas of weakness that may contribute to knee instability.
2. **Consultation with Healthcare Professionals:** If you have existing knee issues or concerns, consult with healthcare professionals, such as physical therapists or orthopedic specialists, to ensure a tailored approach that addresses your specific needs.
3. **Warm-up Routine:** Begin each strength-building session with a comprehensive warm-up routine. Engage in light cardiovascular exercises, dynamic stretches, and joint mobilization to prepare your muscles and joints for the upcoming activities.
4. **Quadriceps Strengthening Exercises:** Target the quadriceps with exercises like leg extensions, squats, and lunges. Ensure proper form and start with a manageable resistance, gradually increasing as your strength improves.
5. **Hamstring Strengthening Exercises:** Strengthen the hamstrings through exercises such as hamstring curls, deadlifts,

and stability ball exercises. Focus on controlled movements and proper technique to avoid unnecessary strain on the knees.

6. **Gluteal Muscle Activation:** Incorporate exercises that activate the gluteal muscles, including bridges, hip thrusts, and lateral leg raises. Strong glutes contribute to hip stability, which, in turn, supports the alignment and function of the knees.

7. **Calf Strengthening Exercises:** Strengthen the calf muscles with exercises like calf raises and heel drops. These exercises help improve the control and stability of the lower leg, reducing the impact on the knee joint during weight-bearing activities.

8. **Balance and Proprioception Training:** Integrate balance and proprioception exercises to improve overall stability. This includes single-leg stands, balance board exercises, and stability ball drills. These activities enhance joint awareness and control.

9. **Flexibility Exercises:** While building strength is crucial, maintaining flexibility is equally important. Include dynamic and static stretching exercises to improve the flexibility of the muscles surrounding the knee joint.

10. **Progressive Resistance Training:** Gradually increase the resistance and intensity of your strength training exercises as your muscles adapt and become stronger. This progressive approach minimizes the risk of overexertion and allows for steady improvement.

11. **Core Strengthening:** Strengthen the core muscles to provide a stable foundation for the entire body. Core exercises such as planks, Russian twists, and bicycle crunches contribute to overall stability and reduce stress on the knees.

12. **Functional Training:** Incorporate functional exercises that mimic real-life movements. This includes activities like step-ups, squats, and lunges, which enhance the coordination and strength of the muscles involved in everyday activities.

13. **Rest and Recovery:** Allow adequate time for rest and recovery between strength-training sessions. Muscles need time to repair and adapt to the demands of training, promoting overall resilience and preventing overuse injuries.

14. **Consistency and Patience:** Building muscular support for knee stability is a gradual process that requires consistency and patience. Stay committed to your strength-building routine, and recognize that positive changes may take time.

8. MINDFUL MOVEMENT

Low-Impact Exercises for Knee Pain Relief

Embarking on the journey of knee joint pain recovery requires a holistic approach that encompasses various facets of physical well-being. Among the key components of this comprehensive plan is the incorporation of mindful movement – low-impact exercises designed to alleviate knee pain while promoting overall joint health. In this article, we will explore the importance of mindful movement and provide a step-by-step guide to low-impact exercises as part of the book "Flex and Thrive: A Step-by-Step Plan for Knee Joint Pain Recovery."

Understanding Knee Pain:

Knee pain is a common ailment that can result from various factors, including injury, overuse, or degenerative conditions like osteoarthritis. The knee joint, being a weight-bearing joint, is susceptible to wear and tear, making it crucial to adopt exercise regimens that prioritize pain relief without exacerbating existing issues. Mindful movement, characterized by low-impact exercises, is a gentle yet effective approach to maintaining joint flexibility, reducing inflammation, and promoting overall knee health.

Benefits of Mindful Movement for Knee Pain:

1. **Gentle on Joints:** Low-impact exercises minimize stress on the knee joints, making them suitable for individuals with existing pain or discomfort. The controlled and deliberate movements reduce the risk of exacerbating injuries.

2. **Improved Range of Motion:** Mindful movement focuses on gentle stretches and controlled motions that contribute to improved range of motion. This is particularly beneficial for individuals experiencing stiffness or reduced mobility in the knees.

3. **Enhanced Joint Lubrication:** The rhythmic and deliberate nature of mindful movement exercises encourages the production and distribution of synovial fluid, which lubricates the joints. This lubrication is crucial for reducing friction and maintaining joint health.

4. **Strengthening Supporting Muscles:** Low-impact exercises target the muscles around the knee, such as the quadriceps, hamstrings, and calf muscles. Strengthening these supporting muscles is essential for providing stability and reducing strain on the knee joint.

5. **Mind-Body Connection:** Mindful movement emphasizes the mind-body connection, encouraging individuals to be present and aware of their movements. This heightened awareness can lead to improved posture, better alignment, and reduced stress on the knees.

Step-by-Step Guide to Mindful Movement for Knee Pain Relief:

1. **Consultation with Healthcare Professionals:** Before beginning any exercise program, especially if you are experiencing knee pain, it is crucial to consult with healthcare professionals such as physical therapists or orthopedic specialists. They can provide personalized recommendations based on your specific condition.

2. **Warm-Up Routine:** Start each session with a gentle warm-up routine to prepare your muscles and joints for exercise. This may include light cardiovascular activities like walking or stationary cycling, as well as dynamic stretches for the lower body.

3. **Seated Leg Lifts (Quadriceps Activation):** Sit on a sturdy chair with your back straight and feet flat on the floor. Lift one

leg straight in front of you, keeping it parallel to the ground. Hold for a moment, then lower it back down. Repeat with the other leg. This exercise targets the quadriceps and helps improve strength and stability.

4. **Standing Calf Raises:** Stand with your feet hip-width apart, near a support for balance if needed. Lift your heels off the ground, rising onto the balls of your feet. Lower your heels back down. This exercise engages the calf muscles, contributing to overall lower limb strength.

5. **Wall Squats:** Stand with your back against a wall and your feet hip-width apart. Slide down the wall into a seated position, ensuring your knees are directly above your ankles. Hold for a few seconds, then slowly rise back up. Wall squats help strengthen the quadriceps and glutes.

6. **Stationary Lunges:** Take a step forward with one foot, lowering your body into a lunge position. Ensure your front knee is directly above your ankle. Push back to the starting position and repeat on the other leg. Stationary lunges target the quadriceps, hamstrings, and glutes.

7. **Seated Knee Extensions:** Sit on a chair with your back straight and feet flat on the floor. Extend one leg straight out in front of you, then lower it back down. Repeat with the other leg. This exercise focuses on the quadriceps and can be adjusted based on your comfort level.

8. **Leg Press (Resistance Band):** Secure a resistance band around a sturdy anchor and sit with your legs extended in front of you. Press your legs against the resistance band, engaging your quadriceps. This exercise provides resistance for muscle strengthening without putting excessive strain on the knees.

9. **Gentle Yoga:** Incorporate gentle yoga poses that focus on stretching and strengthening the lower body. Poses like the child's pose, cat-cow, and downward dog can enhance flexibility and promote relaxation in the knee joints.

10. **Water Aerobics:** Consider low-impact exercises in the water, such as water aerobics or swimming. The buoyancy of the water

reduces the impact on the joints while providing resistance for muscle strengthening.

11. **Tai Chi:** Tai Chi is a mind-body practice that involves slow, flowing movements. It promotes balance, flexibility, and overall joint health. Tai Chi can be adapted to various fitness levels and is well-suited for individuals with knee pain.

12. **Pilates:** Pilates focuses on core strength and stability, making it an excellent choice for individuals with knee issues. Incorporate Pilates exercises that emphasize controlled movements and engage the muscles around the knees.

13. **Cool-Down Routine:** Conclude each session with a thorough cool-down routine to promote relaxation and flexibility. Include static stretches for the lower body, focusing on the quadriceps, hamstrings, calves, and hip flexors.

14. **Mindful Breathing and Meditation:** Dedicate a few minutes to mindful breathing and meditation. This practice can help reduce stress, improve mental focus, and enhance the mind-body connection.

Tips for Incorporating Mindful Movement into Your Routine:

1. **Listen to Your Body:** Pay attention to how your body responds to each exercise. If you experience pain or discomfort, modify the movement or consult with a healthcare professional.

2. **Gradual Progression:** Start with a level of intensity and duration that feels comfortable and gradually progress as your strength and endurance improve. Avoid overexertion to prevent injuries.

3. **Consistency is Key:** Consistency is crucial for reaping the benefits of mindful movement. Aim for regular sessions, even if they are shorter in duration, to establish a routine that supports knee pain relief.

4. **Hydration and Nutrition:** Stay hydrated and maintain a well-balanced diet to support overall joint health. Proper nutrition contributes to the strength and resilience of the muscles surrounding the knees.

5. **Incorporate Variety:** Mix and match different low-impact exercises to keep your routine interesting and target various muscle groups. This variety also prevents overuse injuries.
6. **Rest and Recovery:** Allow your body sufficient time for rest and recovery between mindful movement sessions. Adequate rest is crucial for muscle repair and overall recovery.

9.FLEXIBILITY FUNDAMENTALS

Stretching Techniques for Increased Mobility

I n the pursuit of knee joint pain recovery, the role of flexibility cannot be overstated. Flexibility not only aids in preventing injuries but also contributes significantly to overall joint health and mobility. As part of the comprehensive guide laid out in the book "Flex and Thrive: A Step-by-Step Plan for Knee Joint Pain Recovery," this article will delve into the fundamentals of flexibility, focusing on stretching techniques that enhance mobility while addressing knee pain.

Understanding the Importance of Flexibility:

Flexibility refers to the ability of muscles and joints to move through their full range of motion. For the knees, flexibility is paramount in maintaining smooth and pain-free movements. A lack of flexibility can lead to increased stress on the knee joints, contributing to discomfort, stiffness, and a heightened risk of injuries. Incorporating targeted stretching techniques into your routine can alleviate these issues and promote resilience in the knee joints.

Benefits of Flexibility for Knee Health:

1. **Reduced Joint Stiffness:** Flexible muscles and joints ensure a greater range of motion, reducing stiffness in the knee joint.

This is particularly crucial for individuals experiencing discomfort or tightness.

2. **Enhanced Joint Lubrication:** Stretching promotes the production and distribution of synovial fluid, which lubricates the joints. Proper lubrication is essential for minimizing friction and supporting smooth movements in the knees.

3. **Improved Posture and Alignment:** Flexible muscles contribute to better posture and alignment, reducing unnecessary stress on the knees. Proper alignment is instrumental in preventing uneven wear and tear on joint surfaces.

4. **Prevention of Overuse Injuries:** Overuse injuries can result from repetitive movements that strain the same muscle groups. Flexibility training helps distribute the workload across different muscles, preventing overuse and reducing the risk of injuries.

5. **Better Blood Circulation:** Stretching increases blood flow to the muscles and joints, facilitating nutrient delivery and waste removal. Improved circulation contributes to the overall health of the knee tissues.

Step-by-Step Guide to Stretching Techniques for Increased Mobility:

1. **Consultation with Healthcare Professionals:** Before engaging in any flexibility or stretching program, especially if you are dealing with knee pain, it is essential to consult with healthcare professionals such as physical therapists or orthopedic specialists. They can provide insights into your specific condition and recommend suitable stretches.

2. **Warm-Up Routine:** Always begin your flexibility routine with a thorough warm-up to prepare your muscles and joints for stretching. This can include light cardiovascular exercises like jogging or jumping jacks, as well as dynamic stretches that mimic the movements you'll be performing.

3. **Static Stretching:** Static stretching involves holding a stretch for a prolonged period, typically 15-30 seconds. Focus on major

muscle groups surrounding the knees, including:

- **Quadriceps Stretch:** Stand with one foot bent at the knee and bring your heel towards your buttocks. Hold your ankle with your hand, feeling the stretch in the front of your thigh.
- **Hamstring Stretch:** Sit on the floor with one leg extended and the other bent so the sole of your foot is against the inner thigh of the extended leg. Reach towards your toes, feeling the stretch in the back of your thigh.
- **Calf Stretch:** Stand facing a wall with one foot forward and one foot back. Keep the back leg straight, bend the front knee, and lean towards the wall, feeling the stretch in the calf of the back leg.
- **Inner Thigh Stretch:** Sit on the floor with your legs extended to the sides. Gently lean forward, reaching towards the floor, and feel the stretch along the inner thighs.

4. **Dynamic Stretching:** Dynamic stretching involves controlled, repetitive movements that take your joints through their full range of motion. Examples of dynamic stretches for the knees include:

- **Leg Swings:** Hold onto a stable surface and swing one leg forward and backward in a controlled manner. Repeat on the other leg.
- **Knee Circles:** While seated or standing, gently rotate your knees in a circular motion, first clockwise and then counterclockwise.
- **Walking Lunges:** Take exaggerated steps forward, lowering your body into a lunge position with each step. Keep the movements controlled and fluid.
- **High Knees:** Stand and bring your knees towards your chest in a marching motion. This dynamic stretch engages the hip flexors and quads.

5. **Foam Rolling:** Incorporate foam rolling into your routine to release tension in the muscles and fascia surrounding the knees. Focus on rolling the quadriceps, hamstrings, calves, and IT

band. Apply gentle pressure and adjust based on your comfort level.

6. **Yoga for Knee Flexibility:** Yoga offers a holistic approach to flexibility, combining stretching with breath control and mindfulness. Poses like Downward Dog, Warrior I and II, and Child's Pose can enhance flexibility while promoting relaxation.

7. **Pilates for Core and Leg Strength:** Pilates incorporates controlled movements that target the core and leg muscles. Strengthening these areas contributes to overall stability and complements flexibility training.

8. **Tai Chi for Fluid Movements:** Tai Chi is a mind-body practice characterized by slow, flowing movements. It enhances flexibility, balance, and coordination while being gentle on the joints.

9. **Resistance Band Exercises:** Use resistance bands to add gentle resistance to your stretches. For example, wrap a band around your foot and gently pull it towards your buttocks to enhance the quadriceps stretch.

10. **Balancing Exercises:** Balance exercises, such as single-leg stands or balancing on one leg while performing dynamic movements, engage the muscles around the knee and promote stability.

11. **Cool-Down Routine:** Conclude each stretching session with a cool-down routine to relax the muscles. Include static stretches and deep breathing exercises to facilitate muscle recovery.

Tips for Incorporating Stretching Techniques into Your Routine:

1. **Consistency is Key:** Make stretching a regular part of your routine, aiming for at least 2-3 sessions per week. Consistency is crucial for seeing improvements in flexibility.

2. **Gradual Progression:** Start with gentle stretches and gradually progress to more advanced poses. Avoid pushing yourself too hard, especially if you are new to stretching or dealing with knee pain.

3. **Listen to Your Body:** Pay attention to how your body responds to each stretch. If you experience pain or discomfort beyond mild stretching sensations, ease off and reassess the technique.
4. **Individualized Approach:** Tailor your stretching routine to address your specific needs and limitations. If you have existing knee issues, consult with healthcare professionals to ensure a safe and effective stretching program.
5. **Breath Awareness:** Incorporate mindful breathing into your stretching routine. Deep, controlled breaths can help relax the muscles and enhance the mind-body connection.
6. **Posture and Alignment:** Focus on maintaining proper posture and alignment during stretches. Improper form can contribute to strain and diminish the effectiveness of the stretch.
7. **Hydration and Nutrition:** Stay hydrated and maintain a well-balanced diet to support muscle health. Proper nutrition contributes to the effectiveness of stretching by providing the necessary nutrients for muscle function.
8. **Variety in Stretching Techniques:** Mix and match different stretching techniques to target various muscle groups. This variety prevents boredom and ensures comprehensive flexibility training.

10. PAIN MANAGEMENT STRATEGIES

From Ice Packs to Mindful Breathing

In the pursuit of knee joint pain recovery, effective pain management strategies play a pivotal role in enhancing the overall well-being of individuals. The book "Flex and Thrive: A Step-by-Step Plan for Knee Joint Pain Recovery" recognizes the importance of addressing pain as an integral part of the healing process. This article will comprehensively explore various pain management strategies, ranging from traditional approaches like ice packs to mindfulness techniques such as mindful breathing, providing a holistic guide for individuals on the path to knee joint pain relief.

Understanding Knee Joint Pain:

Knee joint pain can stem from a variety of causes, including injuries, overuse, or degenerative conditions like osteoarthritis. Regardless of the origin, managing pain is a crucial aspect of the recovery process. Pain not only affects physical well-being but can also have a significant impact on mental and emotional health. Therefore, a multifaceted approach to pain management is essential to address the diverse aspects of knee joint pain.

Common Causes of Knee Joint Pain:

1. **Osteoarthritis:** A degenerative joint disease characterized by the breakdown of cartilage, leading to pain, stiffness, and

reduced mobility.

2. **Injuries:** Traumatic injuries, such as ligament sprains, meniscus tears, or fractures, can result in acute or chronic knee pain.
3. **Overuse:** Repetitive stress on the knee joint, often seen in athletes or individuals engaged in activities that involve frequent knee movement, can lead to overuse injuries and pain.
4. **Tendonitis:** Inflammation of the tendons around the knee, causing pain, swelling, and discomfort.
5. **Bursitis:** Inflammation of the bursae, small sacs filled with fluid that cushion the joints, resulting in pain and swelling.

Step-by-Step Pain Management Strategies:

1. **Consultation with Healthcare Professionals:** Before implementing any pain management strategy, it is essential to consult with healthcare professionals, such as orthopedic specialists or pain management specialists. They can provide a thorough assessment of your condition and recommend personalized strategies based on the specific causes of your knee joint pain.
2. **R.I.C.E. Protocol (Rest, Ice, Compression, Elevation):** This classic protocol is effective for managing acute injuries and reducing inflammation:
   - **Rest:** Allow the injured knee to rest and avoid activities that may exacerbate the pain.
   - **Ice:** Apply ice packs to the affected area for 15-20 minutes every 2-3 hours to reduce swelling.
   - **Compression:** Use compression bandages to provide support and minimize swelling.
   - **Elevation:** Elevate the injured knee above heart level to further reduce swelling.
3. **Medication:** Over-the-counter or prescription medications may be recommended for pain relief and inflammation reduction. Nonsteroidal anti-inflammatory drugs (NSAIDs), acetaminophen, or prescribed medications can be considered under the guidance of healthcare professionals.

4. **Physical Therapy:** Physical therapy is a valuable tool for managing knee pain. Therapists can design tailored exercise programs to strengthen muscles, improve flexibility, and address specific issues contributing to knee pain.
5. **Topical Analgesics:** Creams, gels, or patches containing analgesic ingredients like menthol or NSAIDs can be applied topically to the affected area for localized pain relief.
6. **Bracing and Support:** Depending on the nature of the knee issue, braces or supports may be recommended to provide stability, reduce strain, and alleviate pain during movement.
7. **Heat Therapy:** Heat therapy, through hot packs or warm baths, can help relax muscles and increase blood flow to the affected area, promoting healing and pain relief.
8. **Acupuncture:** Acupuncture, an ancient Chinese practice involving the insertion of thin needles into specific points on the body, is believed to stimulate energy flow and alleviate pain.
9. **Massage Therapy:** Massage can help reduce muscle tension, improve circulation, and promote relaxation, contributing to pain relief in individuals with knee joint pain.
10. **Mindful Breathing and Relaxation Techniques:** Mindfulness practices, such as mindful breathing, meditation, and guided imagery, can help manage pain by promoting relaxation and reducing stress.
11. **Cognitive Behavioral Therapy (CBT):** CBT is a therapeutic approach that helps individuals identify and change negative thought patterns and behaviors related to pain, fostering a healthier mindset.
12. **Low-Impact Exercise:** Engaging in low-impact exercises like swimming or cycling can promote joint mobility and strengthen supporting muscles, contributing to pain management.
13. **Weight Management:** Maintaining a healthy weight is crucial for managing knee joint pain, as excess weight places additional stress on the joints. A balanced diet and regular exercise contribute to weight management.
14. **Joint Injections:** In some cases, healthcare professionals may recommend injections of corticosteroids or hyaluronic acid

directly into the knee joint to reduce inflammation and provide pain relief.

15. **Electrotherapy:** Modalities like transcutaneous electrical nerve stimulation (TENS) or ultrasound may be used in physical therapy settings to alleviate pain through the application of electrical currents or sound waves.

16. **Regenerative Medicine:** Emerging treatments, such as platelet-rich plasma (PRP) or stem cell therapy, aim to promote tissue healing and reduce inflammation, offering potential benefits for individuals with knee joint pain.

17. **Support Groups and Counseling:** Emotional well-being is integral to pain management. Joining support groups or seeking counseling can provide a platform for sharing experiences and coping strategies.

18. **Adaptive Devices:** For individuals with chronic knee issues, adaptive devices like canes or orthopedic footwear may be recommended to improve stability and reduce strain on the knees during daily activities.

In-Depth Exploration of Pain Management Strategies:

1. **Rest and Activity Modification:** Rest is crucial for allowing the injured or inflamed tissues to heal. Activity modification involves adjusting your daily activities to minimize stress on the knees. This may include avoiding high-impact exercises, using assistive devices, or altering movement patterns.

2. **Ice Packs and Cold Therapy:** The application of ice packs or cold therapy is a widely used method to reduce inflammation and numb pain. Cold therapy constricts blood vessels, limiting blood flow to the affected area and decreasing swelling.

   - **Proper Ice Pack Application:** Use a cold pack wrapped in a thin cloth to avoid direct contact with the skin. Apply for 15-20 minutes, allowing adequate breaks between sessions.

3. **Compression Bandages:** Compression bandages provide support to the injured area, helping reduce swelling and

promoting joint stability. Ensure the bandage is snug but not too tight, and remove it if you experience numbness or tingling.

4. **Elevation:** Elevating the affected leg above heart level assists in reducing swelling by encouraging the drainage of excess fluid. Use pillows to support the leg while resting.

5. **Medication Management:** Medications, both over-the-counter and prescription, can play a significant role in pain management. NSAIDs, such as ibuprofen or naproxen, reduce inflammation, while acetaminophen provides pain relief without anti-inflammatory properties. Consult with healthcare professionals to determine the most suitable option for your specific needs.

6. **Physical Therapy and Exercise:** Physical therapy involves targeted exercises to strengthen supporting muscles, improve joint mobility, and address biomechanical issues contributing to knee pain. A tailored exercise program may include:

   - **Quad Sets:** Contract the quadriceps muscles, hold for a few seconds, and then relax. Repeat to strengthen the quadriceps.
   - **Hamstring Curls:** While lying on your stomach, bend your knee and bring your heel towards your buttocks. This exercise targets the hamstrings.
   - **Leg Raises:** While lying on your back, lift one leg at a time, keeping it straight. This exercise strengthens the hip flexors and quadriceps.
   - **Calf Raises:** Rise onto the balls of your feet, lifting your heels off the ground. This exercise targets the calf muscles.
   - **Seated Knee Extensions:** Sit on a chair with your back straight and extend one leg straight out in front of you. Hold for a few seconds, then lower it back down. Repeat on the other leg to engage the quadriceps.

7. **Topical Analgesics:** Topical analgesics, available in various forms such as creams, gels, or patches, offer localized pain relief. These products may contain ingredients like menthol,

camphor, or NSAIDs. Apply as directed, avoiding broken or irritated skin.

8. **Bracing and Support:** Knee braces or supports can provide stability and alleviate pain by reducing strain on the affected area. Ensure proper fitting and consult with healthcare professionals for guidance on the most suitable type of brace for your condition.

9. **Heat Therapy:** Heat therapy, using hot packs or warm baths, is beneficial for relaxing muscles and increasing blood flow to the affected area. It is particularly effective for chronic pain or stiffness. Apply heat for 15-20 minutes at a time.

   - **Moist Heat vs. Dry Heat:** Moist heat, such as a warm towel or hot bath, can penetrate tissues more effectively than dry heat. Experiment with both to determine which provides better relief for your knee pain.

10. **Acupuncture:** Acupuncture involves the insertion of thin needles into specific points on the body to stimulate energy flow and promote healing. While research on its efficacy is ongoing, some individuals find relief from knee pain through acupuncture sessions.

11. **Massage Therapy:** Massage therapy can help release tension in muscles surrounding the knee, reduce stiffness, and improve circulation. Choose a licensed massage therapist with experience in treating individuals with knee pain.

12. **Mindful Breathing and Relaxation Techniques:** Mindfulness practices, including mindful breathing and relaxation techniques, can be powerful tools for managing pain. These practices promote a state of calm, reduce stress, and shift focus away from the sensation of pain.

- **Mindful Breathing Exercise:** Sit or lie down comfortably. Inhale deeply through your nose, counting to four. Exhale slowly through your mouth, counting to six. Focus your attention on the breath, allowing it to bring a sense of relaxation.

13. **Cognitive Behavioral Therapy (CBT):** CBT is a therapeutic approach that addresses the connection between thoughts, feelings, and behaviors. In the context of pain management, CBT helps individuals develop coping strategies, challenge negative thought patterns, and improve overall well-being.

- **Journaling:** Keep a pain journal to track patterns, identify triggers, and note the impact of pain on your daily life. This can provide valuable insights for CBT and other therapeutic approaches.

14. **Low-Impact Exercise:** Engaging in low-impact exercises can promote joint mobility, strengthen supporting muscles, and contribute to overall pain management. Consider activities like swimming, cycling, or walking, which are gentle on the knees.

- **Swimming:** Swimming provides a full-body workout with minimal impact on the joints. The buoyancy of water supports the body, making it an excellent option for individuals with knee pain.
- **Cycling:** Cycling, whether on a stationary bike or outdoors, is a low-impact exercise that strengthens the muscles around the knee joint.

15. **Weight Management:** Maintaining a healthy weight is essential for managing knee joint pain, as excess weight places additional stress on the joints. A combination of a balanced diet and regular exercise supports weight management.

- **Nutritional Guidance:** Consult with a nutritionist or healthcare professional for personalized dietary recommendations. A diet rich in anti-inflammatory foods, such as fruits, vegetables, and omega-3 fatty acids, may benefit individuals with knee pain.

16. **Joint Injections:** Injections of corticosteroids or hyaluronic acid directly into the knee joint can provide targeted relief for individuals with inflammatory conditions. These injections aim to reduce inflammation and improve joint function.

17. **Electrotherapy:** Modalities like TENS and ultrasound, commonly used in physical therapy settings, apply electrical currents or sound waves to the affected area. These therapies may help alleviate pain and promote healing.

18. **Regenerative Medicine:** Emerging treatments like PRP or stem cell therapy involve using the body's natural healing processes to address tissue damage and inflammation. While research is ongoing, these treatments show promise for individuals with knee joint pain.

19. **Support Groups and Counseling:** Emotional support is integral to pain management. Joining support groups or seeking counseling can provide a platform for sharing experiences, receiving guidance, and learning coping strategies.

- **Peer Support:** Connecting with others who share similar experiences can provide validation, encouragement, and practical tips for managing the emotional impact of chronic pain.

20. **Adaptive Devices:** For individuals with chronic knee issues, adaptive devices such as canes or orthopedic footwear may be recommended to improve stability and reduce strain on the knees during daily activities.

- **Orthopedic Shoes:** Consider footwear with proper arch support and cushioning to promote comfort and reduce pressure on the knees. Consult with healthcare professionals for recommendations.

In-Depth Exploration of Mindful Breathing and Relaxation Techniques:

Mindful breathing and relaxation techniques play a crucial role in pain management by promoting a state of calm and reducing stress. These practices go beyond the physical aspects of pain, addressing the emotional and psychological components that can intensify discomfort. Incorporating mindful breathing into your routine can contribute to a holistic approach to knee joint pain relief.

1. **Mindful Breathing:** Mindful breathing, also known as diaphragmatic or deep breathing, involves intentional focus on the breath to bring about a sense of calm and relaxation. It can be practiced in various positions – sitting, lying down, or even standing – depending on comfort.

   - **Step-by-Step Mindful Breathing:** a. Find a quiet and comfortable space. b. Sit or lie down in a relaxed position. c. Place one hand on your chest and the other on your abdomen. d. Inhale slowly through your nose, allowing your abdomen to expand as you fill your lungs with air. e. Exhale slowly through your mouth, feeling your abdomen contract. f. Continue this rhythmic breathing, focusing your attention on the sensations of each breath. g. If your mind wanders, gently bring your focus back to the breath.
   - **Benefits of Mindful Breathing:**
     - Calms the nervous system
     - Reduces muscle tension
     - Enhances oxygen flow to the body
     - Promotes mental clarity and focus

2. **Guided Imagery:** Guided imagery involves using your imagination to create calming mental images or scenarios. This technique helps redirect your attention away from pain and stress, fostering a positive and relaxed state of mind.

   - **Guided Imagery Script:** a. Close your eyes and take a few deep breaths. b. Imagine a serene and peaceful place, such as a beach, forest, or meadow.

c. Visualize the details – the colors, sounds, and sensations of this peaceful environment. d. Engage your senses by imagining the warmth of the sun, the sound of gentle waves, or the rustling of leaves. e. Allow yourself to immerse in this calming imagery, letting go of tension and stress. f. Whenever you feel ready, slowly bring your awareness back to the present moment.

- **Benefits of Guided Imagery:**
  - Shifts focus away from pain
  - Promotes relaxation and stress reduction
  - Enhances positive emotions and mental well-being

3. **Progressive Muscle Relaxation (PMR):** PMR involves systematically tensing and then relaxing different muscle groups to release tension and promote relaxation. This technique can be particularly effective for individuals experiencing muscle stiffness or tightness.

- **Step-by-Step PMR:** a. Find a quiet space and get into a comfortable position. b. Start with your toes, tensing the muscles for a few seconds, then releasing the tension completely. c. Move gradually through each muscle group, working your way up the body – feet, calves, thighs, abdomen, chest, arms, neck, and face. d. As you tense and release each muscle group, focus on the sensations of tension and relaxation.

- **Benefits of PMR:**
  - Relieves muscle tension and tightness
  - Promotes overall relaxation
  - Increases body awareness and mindfulness

4. **Body Scan Meditation:** Body scan meditation involves directing focused attention to different parts of the body, bringing awareness to sensations, and releasing tension. This practice enhances mindfulness and can be adapted to specific areas experiencing pain.

- **Guided Body Scan:** a. Lie down in a comfortable position. b. Close your eyes and take a few deep breaths. c. Begin to shift your attention to your toes. Notice any sensations – warmth, tingling, or tension. d. Gradually move your focus up through each part of the body, scanning for sensations and gently releasing tension. e. Continue until you reach the top of your head.

- **Benefits of Body Scan Meditation:**
    - Heightens body awareness
    - Encourages relaxation and stress reduction
    - Cultivates a mindful connection with the body

5. **Breath Awareness Meditation:** Breath awareness meditation involves observing the natural flow of your breath without attempting to control it. This practice promotes mindfulness, helping to anchor your attention in the present moment.

    - **Breath Awareness Exercise:** a. Sit comfortably with a straight spine. b. Close your eyes and bring your attention to your breath. c. Notice the sensation of each inhalation and exhalation. d. If your mind wanders, gently redirect your focus to the breath. e. Continue this mindful awareness for a few minutes.
    - **Benefits of Breath Awareness Meditation:**
        - Cultivates present-moment awareness
        - Calms the mind and reduces mental chatter
        - Enhances the mind-body connection

6. **Yoga Nidra:** Yoga Nidra, also known as yogic sleep, is a form of guided meditation that induces a state of deep relaxation. It involves systematically moving attention through different parts of the body while maintaining a sense of awareness.

    - **Yoga Nidra Script:** a. Lie down in a comfortable position. b. Close your eyes and take a few deep breaths. c. Follow the guided instructions, moving your awareness through various body parts. d. Allow your mind to remain alert while your body experiences a profound state of relaxation.
    - **Benefits of Yoga Nidra:**

- Promotes deep relaxation and stress reduction
- Enhances mental clarity and focus
- Facilitates a sense of inner calm and well-being

Integration of Pain Management Strategies:

1. **Personalized Approach:** Pain management is a highly individualized process, and what works for one person may differ for another. Experiment with various strategies and observe how your body responds. Consult with healthcare professionals to tailor an approach that suits your specific needs.
2. **Combination of Strategies:** A holistic approach to pain management often involves combining multiple strategies. For example, you may incorporate physical therapy exercises, ice packs, and mindful breathing into your routine to address both the physical and emotional aspects of knee joint pain.
3. **Consistency and Patience:** Consistency is key when implementing pain management strategies. Results may not be immediate, and it's essential to be patient and persistent. Gradual improvements over time contribute to sustained relief.
4. **Communication with Healthcare Professionals:** Maintain open communication with your healthcare team throughout the pain management process. Provide feedback on the effectiveness of strategies, report any changes in symptoms, and seek guidance on adjustments or additional interventions.
5. **Adaptation to Changing Needs:** As your condition evolves, be prepared to adapt your pain management strategies accordingly. Periodically reassess your routine, considering new developments or challenges, and consult with healthcare professionals for guidance.

11.ADAPTING YOUR LIFESTYLE

Daily Habits for Knee Joint Wellness

In the journey towards knee joint pain recovery, adopting a holistic approach that encompasses daily habits is key to fostering long-term wellness. The book "Flex and Thrive: A Step-by-Step Plan for Knee Joint Pain Recovery" recognizes the significance of incorporating positive lifestyle changes to support knee health. This article explores various daily habits that contribute to knee joint wellness, providing practical insights and guidance for individuals seeking to adapt their lifestyles as part of a comprehensive recovery plan.

Understanding the Impact of Lifestyle on Knee Joint Health:

The lifestyle choices we make on a daily basis have a profound impact on the health and functionality of our knee joints. From the way we move and engage in physical activity to the foods we consume, each decision plays a role in shaping the well-being of our knees. Recognizing the interconnectedness of lifestyle and knee health is a crucial step towards implementing positive changes that promote flexibility, resilience, and pain-free movement.

Common Lifestyle Factors Affecting Knee Joint Health:

1. **Physical Activity Levels:** The type and intensity of physical activity directly influence the strength, flexibility, and stability of the knee joints. Insufficient or excessive exercise can

contribute to issues such as muscle imbalances, joint strain, or overuse injuries.

2. **Nutrition and Diet:** The foods we consume play a vital role in overall joint health. Nutrient-rich, anti-inflammatory diets support the proper functioning of joints, while poor dietary choices can contribute to inflammation, weight gain, and increased stress on the knees.

3. **Weight Management:** Maintaining a healthy weight is crucial for minimizing stress on the knee joints. Excess body weight places additional strain on the knees, contributing to conditions such as osteoarthritis and accelerating joint degeneration.

4. **Posture and Body Mechanics:** Poor posture and incorrect body mechanics during daily activities can lead to imbalances and increased stress on the knee joints. Proper body alignment supports joint stability and reduces the risk of injuries.

5. **Footwear Choices:** The shoes we wear impact the alignment of our lower extremities and, consequently, the health of our knee joints. Supportive and well-fitted footwear can contribute to proper gait and reduce the risk of misalignments.

6. **Stress Management:** Chronic stress can contribute to muscle tension, inflammation, and overall joint discomfort. Implementing stress management techniques is essential for maintaining a balanced and resilient musculoskeletal system.

7. **Hydration:** Proper hydration is vital for joint health as it supports the lubrication of joints and facilitates the transport of nutrients to the cartilage. Inadequate hydration can contribute to stiffness and reduced joint flexibility.

Step-by-Step Guide to Daily Habits for Knee Joint Wellness:

1. **Maintaining an Active Lifestyle:**
   - **Low-Impact Exercises:** Engage in low-impact exercises that promote joint mobility without excessive stress. Activities such as swimming, cycling, and walking are gentle on the knees while providing cardiovascular benefits.

- **Strength Training:** Incorporate strength training exercises that target the muscles surrounding the knee joints. Focus on building strength in the quadriceps, hamstrings, and calf muscles to provide adequate support.
- **Flexibility Exercises:** Integrate regular stretching and flexibility exercises into your routine. Gentle stretches for the quadriceps, hamstrings, and IT band contribute to improved joint mobility and reduced stiffness.
- **Balance and Stability Training:** Enhance balance and stability through specific exercises. This can include single-leg stands, balance exercises on an unstable surface, or incorporating balance challenges into your strength training routine.
- **Guidelines for Physical Activity:**
  - Gradually increase the intensity and duration of exercise.
  - Listen to your body and modify activities if you experience discomfort.
  - Include a variety of exercises to target different muscle groups.

2. **Balanced and Nutrient-Rich Diet:**
- **Anti-Inflammatory Foods:** Include foods rich in anti-inflammatory properties in your diet. This includes fruits, vegetables, fatty fish, nuts, and seeds. These foods can help reduce inflammation and support overall joint health.
- **Omega-3 Fatty Acids:** Incorporate sources of omega-3 fatty acids, such as salmon, flaxseeds, and chia seeds. Omega-3s have anti-inflammatory effects and contribute to the health of joint tissues.
- **Calcium and Vitamin D:** Ensure adequate intake of calcium and vitamin D for bone health. Dairy products, leafy greens, and fortified foods are good sources of these essential nutrients.

- **Hydration:** Drink plenty of water throughout the day to support joint lubrication and overall hydration. Limit the consumption of sugary beverages, as excess sugar can contribute to inflammation.
- **Moderation and Portion Control:** Practice moderation and portion control to maintain a healthy weight. Overeating can lead to weight gain, placing additional stress on the knee joints.

3. **Weight Management:**
   - **Caloric Balance:** Maintain a caloric balance by consuming an appropriate number of calories based on your activity level and metabolism. This helps prevent weight gain that can strain the knee joints.
   - **Healthy Eating Habits:** Cultivate mindful eating habits, such as listening to hunger and fullness cues, and avoiding emotional eating. Focus on the quality of your food choices.
   - **Regular Physical Activity:** Integrate regular physical activity into your routine to support weight management. Consistent exercise contributes to calorie expenditure and promotes overall well-being.

4. **Posture and Body Mechanics:**
   - **Ergonomic Workspaces:** If you have a desk job, ensure your workspace is ergonomically designed to support good posture. Use an adjustable chair, position your computer screen at eye level, and take breaks to stretch and move.
   - **Proper Lifting Techniques:** When lifting objects, use proper lifting techniques to avoid unnecessary strain on the knees. Bend at the knees, keep the object close to your body, and engage your core muscles.
   - **Body Awareness:** Cultivate body awareness by paying attention to your posture during various activities. This includes sitting, standing, walking,

and performing daily tasks. Correcting poor habits can contribute to long-term joint health.

5. **Footwear Choices:**
   - **Supportive Shoes:** Invest in supportive footwear that provides proper arch support and cushioning. Choose shoes that are well-fitted and appropriate for different activities, whether walking, running, or engaging in specific sports.
   - **Regular Shoe Checks:** Regularly check the condition of your shoes and replace them if they show signs of wear. Worn-out shoes may alter your gait and contribute to joint misalignments.
   - **Orthopedic Inserts:** If necessary, consider using orthopedic inserts or insoles to provide additional support and alignment for your feet. Consult with a podiatrist for personalized recommendations.

6. **Stress Management:**
   - **Mindfulness Practices:** Engage in mindfulness practices such as meditation, deep breathing, or yoga to manage stress. These practices promote relaxation and reduce muscle tension that can contribute to knee discomfort.
   - **Time Management:** Prioritize effective time management to reduce stressors in your daily life. Planning and organizing tasks can help create a more balanced and stress-free environment.
   - **Hobbies and Leisure Activities:** Incorporate hobbies and leisure activities that bring joy and relaxation. Whether it's reading, gardening, or spending time in nature, these activities contribute to overall well-being.

7. **Hydration:**
   - **Water Intake:** Drink an adequate amount of water throughout the day to stay hydrated. Proper hydration supports the lubrication of joints and helps maintain the flexibility of connective tissues.

- **Limit Caffeine and Alcohol:** Limit the consumption of caffeinated and alcoholic beverages, as they can contribute to dehydration. Opt for water, herbal teas, and other hydrating options.
- **Infused Water and Hydration Apps:** Enhance your water intake by infusing water with fruits or herbs for added flavor. Consider using hydration apps to track and remind you to drink water regularly.

Integration of Daily Habits for Knee Joint Wellness:

1. **Consistency and Gradual Implementation:** Adopting daily habits for knee joint wellness requires consistency and gradual implementation. Start by incorporating one or two changes at a time to allow for a smoother transition.
2. **Customization for Individual Needs:** Recognize that each individual's needs and circumstances are unique. Tailor the suggested habits to fit your preferences, lifestyle, and any specific health considerations you may have.
3. **Tracking and Monitoring:** Keep a journal to track your progress and monitor how the implemented habits impact your knee health. Note any changes in pain levels, flexibility, or overall well-being.
4. **Consultation with Healthcare Professionals:** Before making significant lifestyle changes, consult with healthcare professionals, such as orthopedic specialists or physical therapists. They can provide personalized guidance based on your specific condition and needs.

12.OVERCOMING SETBACKS

Navigating Challenges on the Path to Recovery

E mbarking on the journey to recover from knee joint pain is a commendable and empowering pursuit. The book "Flex and Thrive: A Step-by-Step Plan for Knee Joint Pain Recovery" recognizes that the road to healing is not always linear, and setbacks are an inevitable part of the process. This article aims to explore the common challenges individuals may face during their knee joint pain recovery and provide guidance on overcoming setbacks. By acknowledging these obstacles and adopting strategies to navigate them, individuals can cultivate resilience, stay motivated, and ultimately thrive with flexible, pain-free knees.

Understanding Setbacks in Knee Joint Pain Recovery:

Recovering from knee joint pain involves addressing various factors, including physical, emotional, and lifestyle components. Setbacks can manifest in different forms, and their impact may vary from temporary discomfort to more significant hurdles. Recognizing the nature of setbacks is essential for developing effective coping mechanisms and strategies to navigate challenges on the path to recovery.

Common Setbacks in Knee Joint Pain Recovery:

1. **Flare-Ups and Increased Pain:** Individuals may experience flare-ups of pain, stiffness, or swelling, particularly during certain activities or changes in weather. These episodes can be disheartening and may temporarily impede progress.
2. **Plateaus in Progress:** Despite consistent efforts, individuals may encounter plateaus in their recovery journey where they perceive a lack of improvement. This can be discouraging and may lead to feelings of frustration or impatience.
3. **Unforeseen Injuries or Complications:** Unforeseen injuries or complications, either related or unrelated to the knee, can disrupt the recovery process. Dealing with additional health challenges may require adjustments to the initial recovery plan.
4. **Emotional Struggles:** The emotional toll of dealing with chronic pain and the challenges of recovery can contribute to feelings of anxiety, depression, or stress. Emotional well-being is integral to the overall recovery process.
5. **Lack of Motivation:** Sustaining motivation throughout the recovery journey can be challenging, especially if progress is slow or if setbacks occur. A lack of motivation may lead to a decline in adherence to recovery strategies.
6. **External Influences:** External factors, such as work demands, family responsibilities, or lifestyle changes, can impact an individual's ability to consistently prioritize their recovery. Balancing various aspects of life becomes crucial.

Strategies for Overcoming Setbacks:

1. **Cultivating Resilience:**
   - **Mindset Shift:** Embrace a growth mindset that views setbacks as opportunities for learning and adaptation. Recognize that setbacks do not define the entire recovery journey but are natural components of the process.
   - **Positive Affirmations:** Incorporate positive affirmations into your daily routine. Remind yourself of your strengths, achievements, and the progress

you've made, reinforcing a positive and resilient mindset.

- **Self-Compassion:** Practice self-compassion by acknowledging the challenges you face without self-blame. Treat yourself with the same kindness and understanding you would offer to a friend experiencing setbacks.
- **Learn from Setbacks:** Reflect on setbacks to identify potential triggers or factors contributing to the challenge. Use this knowledge to refine your recovery plan, making informed adjustments for improved resilience.

2. **Effective Pain Management:**
    - **Consultation with Healthcare Professionals:** If experiencing increased pain or flare-ups, consult with healthcare professionals promptly. They can provide a thorough assessment, adjust your treatment plan, and offer additional strategies for pain management.
    - **R.I.C.E. Protocol:** Revisit the R.I.C.E. protocol (Rest, Ice, Compression, Elevation) to manage acute flare-ups. Adequate rest, ice application, compression, and elevation can help reduce inflammation and alleviate pain.
    - **Medication Adjustment:** If on pain medications, consult with your healthcare provider to assess their effectiveness. Adjustments or changes in medication may be necessary to better address your pain management needs.

3. **Reassessing and Adjusting Goals:**
    - **Realistic Goal Setting:** Evaluate your initial recovery goals and ensure they are realistic and achievable. Adjust timelines and expectations if necessary, allowing for flexibility in the face of setbacks.
    - **Small Achievements Matter:** Celebrate small achievements along the way. Acknowledge progress,

no matter how incremental, as it contributes to building momentum and maintaining a positive outlook.

- **Consultation with Rehabilitation Specialists:** If progress plateaus, consider consulting with rehabilitation specialists, such as physical therapists or orthopedic experts. They can assess your current status and modify your exercise and rehabilitation plan accordingly.

4. **Embracing Emotional Well-Being:**
   - **Professional Support:** Seek support from mental health professionals if emotional struggles become overwhelming. Therapy, counseling, or support groups can provide valuable tools for managing stress, anxiety, or depression.
   - **Mindfulness Practices:** Integrate mindfulness practices, such as meditation or deep breathing exercises, into your routine. These practices can help manage stress, improve emotional well-being, and enhance resilience.
   - **Open Communication:** Communicate openly with friends, family, or support networks about your emotional challenges. Sharing your feelings and experiences fosters understanding and provides a supportive network.

5. **Motivation Renewal:**
   - **Revisit Your "Why":** Reflect on the reasons behind your commitment to recovery. Reconnecting with your "why" can reignite motivation and remind you of the long-term benefits of your efforts.
   - **Set New Milestones:** Establish new, realistic milestones to work towards. Breaking down the recovery journey into smaller, achievable goals can create a sense of accomplishment and maintain motivation.
   - **Variety in Activities:** Introduce variety into your rehabilitation routine. Exploring new exercises or

activities can prevent monotony and keep you engaged in the recovery process.

6. **Balancing External Influences:**
    - **Time Management Strategies:** Implement effective time management strategies to balance recovery efforts with other life demands. Prioritize self-care and recovery activities by creating a schedule that accommodates both.
    - **Communication and Support:** Communicate openly with those around you about your recovery journey. Seek support from friends, family, or colleagues to ensure understanding and collaboration in balancing external influences.
    - **Adaptation to Life Changes:** If external factors bring about significant life changes, such as a new job or relocation, adapt your recovery plan accordingly. Collaborate with healthcare professionals to modify your approach based on the evolving circumstances.

13. BALANCING ACT

Incorporating Cardiovascular Exercise Safely

C ardiovascular exercise, often synonymous with dynamic movement and vitality, plays a pivotal role in overall health. For individuals on the journey to recover from knee joint pain, finding a balance between reaping the cardiovascular benefits and ensuring joint safety becomes a crucial aspect of the rehabilitation process. The book "Flex and Thrive: A Step-by-Step Plan for Knee Joint Pain Recovery" recognizes the significance of cardiovascular exercise in promoting wellness and explores strategies for incorporating it safely into a comprehensive recovery plan. This article delves into the importance of cardiovascular exercise, the potential challenges for individuals with knee joint pain, and practical guidelines for striking a balance between cardiovascular fitness and joint health.

The Importance of Cardiovascular Exercise for Overall Health:

Cardiovascular exercise, also known as aerobic exercise, involves activities that elevate the heart rate and increase oxygen circulation throughout the body. Regular cardiovascular exercise is associated with a myriad of health benefits, both physical and mental. Some key advantages include:

1. **Heart Health:** Cardiovascular exercise strengthens the heart muscle, enhances blood circulation, and improves overall cardiovascular function. It helps lower blood pressure and reduces the risk of heart-related issues.

2. **Weight Management:** Engaging in regular cardiovascular activity contributes to calorie expenditure, supporting weight management and promoting a healthy body composition. Maintaining a healthy weight is crucial for reducing stress on the knee joints.

3. **Improved Respiratory Function:** Aerobic exercise enhances lung capacity and respiratory function. This increased oxygen intake improves endurance, energy levels, and overall vitality.

4. **Mood Enhancement:** Cardiovascular exercise stimulates the release of endorphins, the body's natural mood elevators. This can help alleviate stress, anxiety, and depression, promoting mental well-being.

5. **Joint Mobility:** While certain forms of cardiovascular exercise may pose challenges for individuals with knee joint pain, others, when performed safely, can contribute to joint mobility and flexibility.

Challenges of Cardiovascular Exercise for Individuals with Knee Joint Pain:

Despite the numerous benefits, individuals recovering from knee joint pain may encounter specific challenges when incorporating cardiovascular exercise into their routine. These challenges include:

1. **Impact on Knee Joints:** High-impact exercises, such as running or jumping, can place significant stress on the knee joints, potentially exacerbating pain or causing discomfort. Individuals with knee issues need to be mindful of activities that involve repeated impact.

2. **Risk of Overuse Injuries:** Overuse injuries can occur when engaging in repetitive movements without adequate recovery. Certain cardiovascular exercises may contribute to overuse injuries, particularly if the biomechanics of the movement strain the knees.

3. **Fear of Aggravating Pain:** The fear of exacerbating knee pain or causing further damage can be a significant psychological

barrier to engaging in cardiovascular exercise. This fear may lead individuals to avoid physical activity altogether.

4. **Limited Range of Motion:** Knee joint pain may be accompanied by a limited range of motion. Some cardiovascular exercises may require a range of motion that individuals with knee issues find challenging or uncomfortable.

5. **Adaptation to Individual Conditions:** Every individual's condition is unique, and what works for one person may not be suitable for another. The challenge lies in finding cardiovascular activities that align with individual abilities, limitations, and preferences.

Strategies for Safely Incorporating Cardiovascular Exercise into Knee Joint Pain Recovery:

1. **Consultation with Healthcare Professionals:**
   - **Medical Evaluation:** Before embarking on any cardiovascular exercise routine, individuals with knee joint pain should undergo a thorough medical evaluation. This may include consultations with orthopedic specialists, physical therapists, or rehabilitation experts.
   - **Individualized Recommendations:** Healthcare professionals can provide personalized recommendations based on the specific condition, severity of knee joint pain, and any underlying issues. This guidance ensures that the chosen cardiovascular activities are safe and aligned with the individual's recovery goals.

2. **Low-Impact Cardiovascular Exercises:**
   - **Swimming:** Swimming is a low-impact exercise that provides a full-body workout without placing stress on the knee joints. It enhances cardiovascular fitness, builds muscle strength, and supports joint mobility.
   - **Cycling:** Stationary or recumbent cycling is gentle on the knees and promotes cardiovascular health. Adjust the resistance level based on comfort,

allowing for a customizable and low-impact workout.

- **Elliptical Training:** The elliptical machine provides a low-impact alternative to running. It simulates the motion of running without the jarring impact, making it suitable for individuals with knee joint pain.
- **Rowing:** Rowing engages both the upper and lower body while minimizing impact on the knee joints. It offers an effective cardiovascular workout with the added benefit of strengthening multiple muscle groups.

3. **Gradual Progression and Monitoring:**
    - **Start Slow:** Begin with low-intensity exercises and gradually increase the duration and intensity as tolerance improves. This approach allows the body to adapt and minimizes the risk of overuse injuries.
    - **Listen to Your Body:** Pay attention to signals from your body during and after exercise. If you experience pain, discomfort, or swelling, modify or discontinue the activity and consult with healthcare professionals.
    - **Pacing and Rest:** Incorporate adequate rest and recovery days into your cardiovascular exercise routine. Pacing yourself and allowing for sufficient recovery time are crucial for preventing overuse injuries.

4. **Strength Training for Joint Support:**
    - **Focus on Muscular Support:** Incorporate strength training exercises that target the muscles surrounding the knee joints. Strengthening the quadriceps, hamstrings, and calf muscles provides added support and stability.
    - **Balanced Muscle Development:** Achieve balanced muscle development to avoid muscle imbalances, which can contribute to joint strain. Consult with

fitness professionals or physical therapists for a tailored strength training program.

5. **Joint-Friendly Cardio Classes:**
   - **Water Aerobics:** Water aerobics classes provide a buoyant and supportive environment for cardiovascular exercise. The resistance of the water enhances muscle engagement without stressing the knee joints.
   - **Low-Impact Dance Classes:** Participate in low-impact dance classes that prioritize fluid movements and minimize stress on the knees. Look for classes specifically designed for individuals with joint considerations.
   - **Adapted Cardio Programs:** Explore adapted cardio programs or classes designed for individuals with joint conditions. These programs often incorporate modifications to traditional exercises to make them more joint-friendly.

6. **Mindful Exercise Techniques:**
   - **Proper Form and Alignment:** Pay attention to proper form and body alignment during cardiovascular exercise. Maintaining correct posture reduces the risk of strain on the knees and ensures effective and safe movement.
   - **Range of Motion Awareness:** Be mindful of your range of motion, especially if you have limitations due to knee joint pain. Choose exercises that allow for controlled and comfortable movement without pushing beyond your capabilities.
   - **Mind-Body Connection:** Cultivate a strong mind-body connection during exercise. This awareness helps you respond to your body's signals, adapt as needed, and prevent potential injuries.

7. **Cross-Training Approach:**
   - **Variety of Activities:** Adopt a cross-training approach by incorporating a variety of cardiovascular activities. This not only prevents

boredom but also reduces the risk of overuse injuries associated with repetitive movements.

- **Balanced Exercise Routine:** Include a mix of low-impact aerobic exercises, strength training, and flexibility work in your routine. A balanced exercise regimen supports overall joint health and enhances cardiovascular fitness.

8. **Regular Monitoring and Adjustment:**

- **Reassess Your Routine:** Regularly reassess your cardiovascular exercise routine to ensure it aligns with your evolving needs and recovery progress. Consult with healthcare professionals for guidance on adjustments or modifications.

- **Tracking Progress:** Keep a journal to track your cardiovascular exercise sessions, noting the type, duration, and intensity. Monitoring progress allows you to celebrate achievements and identify areas for improvement.

- **Consultation with Experts:** If facing challenges or uncertainties, consult with fitness professionals, physical therapists, or rehabilitation specialists. Their expertise can provide valuable insights and contribute to the ongoing refinement of your cardiovascular exercise plan.

14.SURGICAL OPTIONS

Exploring and Understanding Knee Interventions

Knee joint pain can be a persistent and challenging condition that significantly impacts daily life. While many individuals find relief through conservative approaches like physical therapy and lifestyle modifications, there are cases where surgical interventions become a necessary step towards achieving optimal knee health. The book "Flex and Thrive: A Step-by-Step Plan for Knee Joint Pain Recovery" recognizes the importance of exploring and understanding surgical options as part of a comprehensive recovery plan. This article delves into various surgical interventions for knee joint issues, providing insights into their purposes, procedures, recovery processes, and considerations for individuals navigating this aspect of their knee health journey.

Section 1: Understanding Knee Anatomy and Common Issues:

1.1 **Anatomy of the Knee Joint:** To comprehend the rationale behind various knee interventions, it's crucial to understand the anatomy of the knee joint. The knee is a complex structure comprising bones, ligaments, tendons, and cartilage. The femur (thigh bone), tibia (shin bone), and patella (kneecap) form the bony components, while ligaments and tendons provide stability and connective support.

1.2 **Common Knee Issues:** Knee joint pain can arise from a variety of conditions, including osteoarthritis, rheumatoid arthritis, meniscus tears, ligament injuries (such as ACL or PCL tears), and patellar dislocation. The severity and nature of the issue often dictate the appropriate surgical intervention.

Section 2: Types of Surgical Interventions:

2.1 **Arthroscopy:** Arthroscopy is a minimally invasive surgical procedure that involves the insertion of a small camera (arthroscope) through tiny incisions in the knee. This allows the surgeon to visualize and diagnose issues, such as meniscus tears or cartilage damage. Arthroscopic procedures are often used for both diagnostic and therapeutic purposes.

2.2 **Meniscus Repair or Partial Meniscectomy:** Meniscus tears are a common knee injury. Depending on the type and location of the tear, surgical options may include repairing the torn meniscus or removing the damaged portion through a partial meniscectomy. The goal is to alleviate pain and restore knee function.

2.3 **Ligament Reconstruction:** Ligament injuries, particularly to the anterior cruciate ligament (ACL) or posterior cruciate ligament (PCL), may require reconstruction. This involves replacing the damaged ligament with a graft, often sourced from the patient's own tissue or a donor. Ligament reconstruction aims to restore stability and prevent further joint damage.

2.4 **Total Knee Replacement (TKR):** Total knee replacement is a major surgical intervention for advanced knee osteoarthritis or severe joint degeneration. The procedure involves replacing the damaged knee joint surfaces with artificial components made of metal and plastic. TKR aims to alleviate pain, improve mobility, and enhance overall knee function.

2.5 **Partial Knee Replacement:** In cases where only one compartment of the knee is affected, partial knee replacement may be considered. This procedure replaces only the damaged portion of the knee joint, preserving the healthy areas. Partial knee replacement is a less invasive option with a quicker recovery compared to total knee replacement.

2.6 **Cartilage Restoration:** Various techniques exist for cartilage restoration, aimed at addressing focal cartilage defects. Procedures like microfracture, autologous chondrocyte implantation (ACI), and matrix-induced autologous chondrocyte implantation (MACI) aim to promote the growth of new, healthy cartilage in the damaged areas.

2.7 **Osteotomy:** Osteotomy involves surgically altering the alignment of the bones around the knee joint. This procedure is typically considered for individuals with early-stage osteoarthritis, aiming to shift weight-bearing forces away from the damaged part of the joint and alleviate symptoms.

Section 3: Considerations and Decision-Making:

3.1 **Patient Evaluation:** Before recommending any surgical intervention, thorough patient evaluation is crucial. This includes a comprehensive examination of the knee joint, imaging studies (such as X-rays and MRI scans), and consideration of the patient's overall health and lifestyle.

3.2 **Conservative Approaches:** While surgical options are valuable tools in addressing knee issues, conservative approaches should be exhausted before considering surgery. Physical therapy, lifestyle modifications, medications, and other non-invasive methods play a significant role in managing knee pain and improving function.

3.3 **Individualized Treatment Plans:** Knee interventions are not one-size-fits-all. Treatment plans should be tailored to the individual, taking into account factors such as age, activity level, overall health, and the specific nature of the knee issue. Shared decision-making between the patient and healthcare team is crucial.

3.4 **Potential Risks and Complications:** All surgical interventions carry inherent risks and potential complications. Patients should be informed about these risks, including infection, blood clots, anesthesia-related issues, and the possibility of incomplete pain relief or functional improvement.

3.5 **Rehabilitation and Recovery:** Understanding the rehabilitation process is essential for individuals considering knee surgery. Physical therapy, post-operative exercises, and adherence to rehabilitation protocols are crucial for a successful recovery and optimal outcomes.

Section 4: Post-Surgery Recovery and Rehabilitation:

4.1 **Immediate Post-Operative Care:** Following knee surgery, immediate post-operative care is focused on managing pain, reducing swelling, and preventing complications. This may involve the use of pain medications, ice therapy, and compression.

4.2 **Physical Therapy:** Physical therapy is a cornerstone of post-surgery recovery. It aims to restore joint mobility, strengthen surrounding muscles, improve flexibility, and enhance overall functional capacity. The type and intensity of physical therapy depend on the specific surgery and the individual's progress.

4.3 **Gradual Resumption of Activities:** Patients should follow a gradual resumption of activities guided by their healthcare team. This may involve transitioning from assisted devices (such as crutches) to full weight-bearing, increasing the range of motion, and incorporating more challenging exercises as tolerated.

4.4 **Long-Term Rehabilitation Goals:** Long-term rehabilitation goals include achieving optimal joint function, minimizing pain, and preventing future issues. Patients are encouraged to actively participate in their recovery by adhering to prescribed exercises, attending follow-up appointments, and communicating with their healthcare team.

Section 5: Lifestyle Considerations After Surgery:

5.1 **Maintaining Joint Health:** Following knee surgery, individuals should adopt lifestyle habits that promote joint health. This includes maintaining a healthy weight, engaging in regular low-impact exercises, and avoiding activities that may place excessive stress on the treated knee.

5.2 **Nutrition and Hydration:** Proper nutrition plays a crucial role in supporting the healing process. Adequate intake of nutrients like vitamin C, vitamin D, and protein is essential for tissue repair and overall joint health. Staying hydrated also contributes to joint lubrication.

5.3 **Regular Monitoring and Follow-Up:** Regular monitoring and follow-up appointments with healthcare professionals are essential for tracking long-term outcomes, addressing any emerging issues, and ensuring continued joint health. Open communication about any concerns or changes in symptoms is encouraged.

15. LIFELONG FLEX AND THRIVE

Sustaining Knee Health for the Long Run

As we journey through life, our knees bear the weight of our experiences, both figuratively and literally. Knee health is a cornerstone of overall well-being, allowing us to engage in a wide range of activities, from daily tasks to sports and recreation. The book "Flex and Thrive: A Step-by-Step Plan for Knee Joint Pain Recovery" recognizes that sustaining knee health is not just about recovery but also about cultivating lifelong habits that promote flexibility, strength, and resilience. This article explores the principles and practices essential for lifelong knee health, providing a comprehensive guide to ensure that individuals not only recover from knee issues but thrive with flexible, pain-free knees throughout their lives.

Section 1: Understanding Lifelong Knee Health:

1.1 **The Importance of Lifelong Knee Health:** Lifelong knee health is not only about preventing and managing pain but also about preserving the integrity and functionality of the knee joints. A proactive approach to knee care contributes to a higher quality of life, enabling individuals to maintain an active and fulfilling lifestyle.

1.2 **Common Challenges in Aging Knees:** As we age, the knees undergo natural wear and tear. Conditions such as osteoarthritis, decreased cartilage thickness, and reduced joint fluid can affect knee function. Understanding these challenges allows for informed decision-making and proactive measures to mitigate potential issues.

Section 2: Physical Activity for Lifelong Knee Health:

2.1 **Low-Impact Exercise for All Ages:** Engaging in regular low-impact exercises is key to promoting lifelong knee health. Activities such as walking, swimming, and cycling provide cardiovascular benefits without placing excessive stress on the knee joints, making them suitable for individuals of all ages.

2.2 **Strength Training for Joint Support:** Incorporating strength training exercises is essential for providing muscular support to the knee joints. Targeting the quadriceps, hamstrings, and calf muscles helps maintain joint stability and prevents imbalances that can contribute to knee issues.

2.3 **Flexibility and Range of Motion Exercises:** Maintaining flexibility is crucial for preserving the range of motion in the knees. Stretching exercises, yoga, and tai chi can enhance flexibility, reduce stiffness, and contribute to overall joint health.

2.4 **Balancing Exercises:** Enhancing balance is a key aspect of preventing falls and minimizing the risk of injuries to the knees, especially in older adults. Simple balancing exercises can be incorporated into daily routines to improve stability.

2.5 **Adapting Exercise Routines Over Time:** As individuals age or experience changes in knee health, adapting exercise routines becomes essential. Customizing activities to accommodate specific needs and modifying intensity based on comfort levels ensures ongoing participation in physical activity.

Section 3: Nutrition and Lifestyle Habits for Lifelong Knee Health:

3.1 **Maintaining a Healthy Weight:** Body weight plays a significant role in knee health. Maintaining a healthy weight reduces the load on the knees, lowering the risk of conditions like osteoarthritis. A balanced diet and regular physical activity contribute to weight management.

3.2 **Nutrient-Rich Diet for Joint Support:** A diet rich in nutrients essential for joint health supports the maintenance of cartilage, ligaments, and other knee structures. Omega-3 fatty acids, antioxidants, vitamin D, and calcium are particularly beneficial for preserving knee function.

3.3 **Hydration for Joint Lubrication:** Staying adequately hydrated is crucial for joint lubrication. Water helps maintain the synovial fluid that cushions the knee joints, promoting smooth movement and reducing friction.

3.4 **Healthy Lifestyle Choices:** Lifestyle habits, such as avoiding smoking and excessive alcohol consumption, contribute to overall health, including knee health. These choices support the body's ability to repair and maintain tissues, fostering optimal joint function.

Section 4: Joint-Friendly Practices in Daily Life:

4.1 **Proper Body Mechanics:** Adopting proper body mechanics in daily activities, such as sitting, standing, and lifting, reduces unnecessary stress on the knees. Maintaining good posture and using ergonomic principles contribute to joint-friendly practices.

4.2 **Footwear Choices:** The choice of footwear significantly impacts knee health. Wearing supportive and comfortable shoes that provide proper arch support and cushioning helps distribute weight evenly, reducing the strain on the knees.

4.3 **Environment Modifications:** Making simple modifications in the home and work environment, such as using handrails, installing ramps, and ensuring well-lit spaces, promotes safety and minimizes the risk of falls or injuries that could impact knee health.

4.4 **Regular Health Check-ups:** Regular health check-ups, including joint assessments, contribute to the early detection of potential knee issues. Timely intervention and preventive measures can help address issues before they escalate.

Section 5: Mental and Emotional Well-Being:

5.1 **Stress Management:** Stress can contribute to muscle tension and exacerbate knee discomfort. Incorporating stress management techniques, such as meditation, deep breathing, or mindfulness, promotes relaxation and overall well-being.

5.2 Mental Health and Physical Activity: The connection between mental health and physical activity is profound. Engaging in regular exercise releases endorphins, contributing to a positive mood and reducing the perception of pain. It also fosters a sense of accomplishment and empowerment.

5.3 Social Connection and Support: Maintaining social connections and seeking support from friends, family, or support groups contributes to emotional well-being. Sharing experiences and challenges fosters a sense of community and resilience in managing knee health.

Section 6: Regular Monitoring and Preventive Measures:

6.1 Regular Joint Assessments: Periodic joint assessments by healthcare professionals help monitor knee health and detect any emerging issues. Individuals with a history of knee problems or those at higher risk should schedule regular check-ups.

6.2 Preventive Measures for Specific Populations: Certain populations, such as athletes, individuals with a family history of knee issues, or those with specific medical conditions, may benefit from targeted preventive measures. This may include customized exercise routines, biomechanical assessments, or additional screening.

6.3 Understanding Warning Signs: Knowledge of warning signs, such as persistent pain, swelling, or changes in mobility, empowers individuals to seek prompt medical attention. Early intervention can prevent the progression of knee issues and improve long-term outcomes.

Section 7: Adapting to Life Changes:

7.1 Life Transitions and Knee Health: Life transitions, such as retirement or changes in physical activity levels, may necessitate adjustments in knee health practices. Adapting to these changes ensures continued well-being and flexibility.

7.2 Consultation with Healthcare Professionals: When facing significant life changes or health challenges, consulting with healthcare professionals provides valuable guidance. Orthopedic specialists, physical therapists, and other experts can offer personalized recommendations based on individual needs.

7.3 Customization for Aging: As individuals age, customization becomes key. Tailoring exercise routines, dietary choices, and lifestyle habits to align with the changing needs of the body supports ongoing knee health.

9 798223 943433